ENGLISH MEDICINE & THE
CAMBRIDGE SCHOOL

ENGLISH MEDICINE & THE CAMBRIDGE SCHOOL

An Inaugural Lecture

BY

W. LANGDON BROWN

M.A., M.D., F.R.C.P.

Regius Professor of Physic in the University of Cambridge

Consulting Physician to St Bartholomew's Hospital, London

CAMBRIDGE
AT THE UNIVERSITY PRESS
1932

CAMBRIDGE
UNIVERSITY PRESS

University Printing House, Cambridge CB2 8BS, United Kingdom

Published in the United States of America by Cambridge University Press, New York

Cambridge University Press is part of the University of Cambridge.

It furthers the University's mission by disseminating knowledge in the pursuit of
education, learning and research at the highest international levels of excellence.

www.cambridge.org
Information on this title: www.cambridge.org/9781107697881

First published 1932
Re-issued 2014

A catalogue record for this publication is available from the British Library

ISBN 978-1-107-69788-1 Paperback

ENGLISH MEDICINE & THE CAMBRIDGE SCHOOL

━━━━━━

I T is just forty years since I listened to an Inaugural Lecture by the Regius Professor of Physic. On that occasion Sir Clifford Allbutt presented a survey of medicine which made a profound impression upon me; its breadth of vision gave me a new conception of what medicine might be.

During his tenure of this Chair, Sir Clifford added both lustre and dignity to it. It was indeed fortunate that during a time of such rapid development of the Medical School of this University, the Chair was occupied by a man of such outstanding distinction, high character and personal charm. His profound learning did not lead him to despise the practical details of his profession. The introduction of the short clinical thermometer in common use, and to a large extent, the hypodermic syringe, we owe to Sir Clifford Allbutt. His successor, Sir Humphry Rolleston, who is endeared to me by innumerable acts of kindness, is fortunately still among us. His scientific and professional attainments are known to all and I do not hesitate to say that there is no man more looked up to and beloved in the medical profession to-day. I imagine that he is the only Regius Professor of Physic who has been an Admiral. He is certainly only the second Regius Professor of Physic to have been also President of the Royal College of Physicians, Glisson having been elected to that office in 1667. Cambridge may well congratulate herself that the finest System of Medicine published in English bears the two names of Allbutt and Rolleston as joint Editors. Among other debts, we owe Sir Humphry gratitude for his recent biographical history of the Cambridge Medical School. My indebtedness to this book will be obvious in the brief résumé I shall presently give of the earlier history of medicine in Cambridge.

But before embarking on that history, I

should like to remind you that it illustrates the curiously spasmodic character of medical progress. Only a day or two after I knew that I was to have the honour of occupying this Chair, I was reading the Inaugural Lecture prepared by Mr Lowes Dickinson, now, alas, no longer with us. His lecture specially attracted me because it illuminated one aspect of my subject. Dickinson posed this question— Greece was the birthplace of Natural Science, and, I might interpolate, of scientific as opposed to magical medicine. Why was it extinguished so early and so completely? Why did it not develop continuously? His own answer was as follows—science is concerned not with goodness or badness but with facts and their interpretation. The change from the study of things to the study of values began before science had established its authority by showing its practical utility. Although it was in Greece that Natural Science was born, Greece became instead the mother of famous systems of ethics. If science had even begun to show its utility, the Romans, who were a practical people, would have fostered such studies, instead of interesting themselves in Epicureanism and Stoicism. But science appeared to them futile. "For this they paid the penalty; for their civilisation perished by a kind of atrophy, and there descended upon the Western world an age of darkness in which nothing remained of the Greek spirit but a gradually ossifying literature and so much of the Graeco-Roman tradition as was embodied in the amalgam of Christian theology. Almost everything that had been discovered and known was forgotten for a thousand years, and what was more, the spirit itself was extinguished."

The modern application of science to life on a tremendous scale is a thing quite new in history. Man's brain cannot adapt itself quickly enough to the material changes of the last 100 years. Our environment is changing faster than ourselves. Lowes Dickinson realised that we too are faced with the dilemma of Graeco-Roman society. To quote him again: "How are we to deal with science? Shall we allow it to destroy us, or shall we destroy it to save ourselves? Neither way seems a good one; but is there not another alternative? There is, clearly, if we would but take it. Our science, we saw, is the product of the Greek spirit; but so is our ethics. In the Graeco-Roman crisis these two movements fought one another, till ethics, in the end, destroyed science. What we have to do is to reconcile the antagonists—to apply ethics to science and science to ethics. That movement, I think, has already begun; and on its success depends the future of civilisation".

To a medical man this point of view is of great interest, for not only does medicine attempt to combine science with ethics in its relief of suffering, but in these latter days is becoming increasingly psychological in its approach to disease while developing its scientific armament as much as possible. Medical science in its broadest aspects, therefore, may well be a pioneer in this reconciling process from which Dickinson hoped for so much.

During those thousand years of darkness of which he speaks, only the Arabs kept a flickering candle alight. Then with the Renaissance came our first opportunity of establishing a school of medicine here. I can never pass through Queens' College without looking up, with a feeling akin to reverence, at Erasmus' tower. There was indeed a beacon. If the Reformation had had Erasmus instead of Luther for its leader what a different story it would have been. But the scholar is no match for the demagogue in an appeal to the herd. However, that is a digression. Where Erasmus comes into my story is that he was accompanied by John Siberch, who began the history of Cambridge printing by establishing a press here in 1521. Eight complete specimens of his printing survive, and as far as we know, the fourth book published by his press in that year was a discourse on Galen by Thomas Linacre. Now Linacre was the founder of English academic medicine. In 1518 he persuaded Henry VIII to constitute the Royal College of

Physicians, and six years later, just eight days before his death, founded lectureships both at Oxford and Cambridge. But while his London enterprise flourished his University gifts were sadly mismanaged for centuries. In 1540 Henry VIII established five Regius Professorships here, that of Physic being one. Sir Humphry Rolleston remarks that although this should have ensured a living school of medicine at Cambridge, the results were most disappointing, for while cultivating the intellectual needs, the University atmosphere was conservatively hostile to those of the body. Here again, is an instance of that antagonism of which Dickinson spoke. Medical students who wished to get real teaching were obliged to seek it elsewhere, as Harvey, Caius and others did at Padua, and none of them, when they came back to England, founded a school at Cambridge. Harvey, for instance, expounded his immortal discovery of the circulation of the blood not in Cambridge, but as Lumleian Lecturer at the College of Physicians.

The treatment meted out to Caius in spite of his munificent benefactions makes painful reading. Glisson, whose name is permanently inscribed for every medical student on the structure of the liver, was the outstanding Regius Professor in the seventeenth century. He held office for 41 years, yet he was largely an absentee. Medical teaching, such as it was, from the birth of the University until the nineteenth century consisted in the reading and expounding of Hippocrates, Galen and Aretaeus, and was devoid of the experimental method in which Harvey could have led the way. And that in spite of the fact that in 1705 Richard Bentley, the turbulent Master of Trinity, over-rode his senior fellows and established a physiological laboratory there, in which Stephen Hales, a member of Corpus Christi (the College to which I now have the honour to belong), and the discoverer of blood pressure, carried out experiments, after a sound training in Newtonian physics. But little else stirred the general stagnation. It is astonishing to learn that even as late as 1870 only two M.D. and seven M.B. degrees were conferred, while in 1877 the four examiners passed five candidates.

Sociologists tell us that the renaissance of a nation is always heralded by the outbreak of an "heroic age". It is generally assumed that it was the advent of George Murray Humphry to Cambridge which led to the rebirth of its medical school, and he certainly was an heroic figure. But Sir Humphry Rolleston points out that the foundations had been quietly laid by John Haviland who was Regius Professor from 1817 to 1851, ably seconded by Sir George Paget who became Regius in 1872. I just remember seeing Sir George Paget in his old age, a frail but distinguished figure. This school owes much to his prophetic vision and untiring effort, just as my other school, St Bartholomew's, is greatly indebted to Sir James Paget. The effect of these two brothers on medical education has been profound and far-reaching. They have been compared with another great pair of brothers, also surgeon and physician respectively, John and William Hunter. It was on the advice of the Paget brothers that George Murray Humphry was brought to Cambridge. A Suffolk man, he was apprenticed at the early age of 16 to the well-known surgeon John Green Crosse at Norwich, and subsequently entered St Bartholomew's Hospital, where he came under the influence of the famous Peter Mere Latham, whose emphatic style of teaching he adopted. On October 31st, 1842, when only 22 years of age, he was elected surgeon to Addenbrooke's, a post he held for 52 years. In less than two months he had obtained permission to deliver clinical lectures there. From 1848 he was responsible for the teaching of anatomy, becoming Professor in 1866. His energy was terrific. In addition to teaching surgery and anatomy, he found time from the demands of a busy practice to pour out a constant stream of papers on anatomical, pathological and surgical subjects, which secured his election as an F.R.S. in 1859. His ambition was to make Cambridge a complete school of medicine, and Addenbrooke's Hospital was largely rebuilt from plans he prepared. On the site where the Leys School now stands, he established a hostel for medical students to enable those of small means to come to the University for the whole of their training. But his very success in drawing students made such a scheme impracticable. There was not, and cannot be, clinical material available for a large number of students, although Addenbrooke's is far more adequate now than then. In 1883 he resigned the Professorship of Anatomy and offered to become Professor of Surgery without stipend, a post he held till his death in 1896 at the age of 76. One can see him now, with his glittering hawk-like eye, ready to pounce on ignorance and sloth, but equally ready to help. A born teacher, he has been described as "magnetic and Socratic"; innumerable anecdotes cluster round his name. One must suffice. "On one occasion a student not remarkable for ability somewhat unexpectedly answered a question correctly, and followed it up by the unwise comment, 'You seem surprised, Professor', only to be discomfited by the prompt retort, 'So was Balaam when his ass spoke'."

Humphry keenly advocated the establishment of a Chair of Physiology, but there were delays. Here again, as in 1705, Trinity College came to the rescue largely owing to the efforts of Coutts-Trotter, and on Huxley's recommendation brought Michael Foster from University College, London, as Praelector and Fellow. No more fortunate choice could have been made. Although at first his only laboratory was a corner of the Philosophical Library, he rapidly gathered a brilliant band of students round him. W. H. Gaskell, who had graduated as a Wrangler, seeing a notice of a lecture to be given by Foster, strolled in to hear it. That determined his future career, with what enormous consequences to English physiology everyone knows. J. N. Langley entered St John's College the year after Foster's arrival, and after gaining a first class in the Natural Sciences Tripos subsequently became his demonstrator. In 1903, he succeeded Sir Michael Foster in the Professorship which had been established in 1883. Gaskell said of Foster, "He was a discoverer of men rather than of facts, and he worked for rather than at physiology". He had an enormous influence in determining the careers of his followers, for he was a supreme judge of men. This triumvirate of Paget, Humphry and Foster was the controlling factor in ensuring success, but we must not forget the part also played by Alexander Macalister. A great anatomist, he took all learning for his province.

And now, the failure at the time of the Renaissance to establish a living school of medicine in Cambridge was at length to be gloriously redeemed. I was not here to see the springtide which followed the long winter, for when I entered in 1889 it was already early summer, but from my teachers I heard much of that swift flowering. This leads me to my main topic—the influence of this later Renaissance on English medicine. I propose to confine myself almost entirely to the influence of the work which was undertaken, completed or initiated during my five years residence, for of this alone have I first-hand knowledge. The words of the old school song resound in my ears, "How will it seem to you, forty years on?" I want to tell you how the achievements of those days seem to me now, and how their influence is still living after an interval of forty years.

First, I will deal with its effect upon modern cardiology. Foster and Dew-Smith had been studying the automatic rhythm of the invertebrate heart. Gaskell, who had been working in Germany with Ludwig on the cardio-vascular system, returned to Cambridge to study the influence of chemical substances on the calibre of the peripheral blood vessels. Finding that the muscles of the arterioles were responsive to other than nervous stimuli, his interest in the heart muscle was aroused by this work of Foster and Dew-Smith. Up to that time, the rhythm of the heart was attributed to the nerve ganglia within that organ. Gaskell showed by a simple experiment that the physiologically disconnected ventricle of the frog's heart would assume an independent rhythm if the pressure within the heart were raised sufficiently to stretch its musculature. To my mind, at that moment, modern cardiology was born, although more than twenty years were to elapse before the clinical applications were made. The subsequent phases of his work are classical, and I need not detail them here. They led him to the conclusion that cardiac rhythm was a property of the heart muscle rather than of the nerve ganglia; a view which in a somewhat modified form, is still held. These results could not be applied to a mammalian heart until muscular continuity between its auricles and ventricles was established by Stanley Kent in 1892, and His described in the following year the node and bundle which usually go by his name. Next, Tawara traced this bundle in more detail, showing that it was continued into certain curious fibres of hitherto unknown significance which Purkinje had described as long ago as 1845.

The interest of the story now shifts from the laboratory to the consulting room. A busy practitioner in Burnley had been laboriously studying for years the forms of cardiac irregularity he found in patients and recording them by means of an instrument he had invented—the polygraph. Needless to say, I mean James Mackenzie. His approach was purely clinical, but he himself once said to me, "The further I go, the more I realise that Gaskell was the man". For in Gaskell's pioneer work he found the explanation of many of his observations on disturbed heart rhythm, particularly, of course, heartblock.

Discovery often has to wait for the invention of new tools. Einthoven's string galvanometer proved to be the tool which opened the door to further discoveries. But much depends on the man who wields the tool, and it required a Sir Thomas Lewis to conquer the new fields that were thus opened to him, by applying the electrocardiograph with a skill, subtlety and accuracy which have commanded the admiration of his contemporaries. Here I will break my self-imposed limits to point out that two pieces of work done here subsequent to my time contributed materially to such conquests. For Lewis found in G. R. Mines' observations on circus movements in muscle the key to the mechanism of auricular fibrillation, while A. V. Hill's demonstration that the energy developed by muscular contraction was proportional to its previous stretching enabled Starling to enunciate "the law of the heart" in his memorable Linacre Lecture of 1915. We may therefore fairly claim that the influence of Cambridge on modern cardiology has been profound.

I should like to turn next to the Sympathetic Nervous System, or to use a more inclusive term, the Involuntary Nervous System. The elucidation of this will always remain one of the greatest achievements of the Cambridge School. There cannot be many physicians still practising who actually worked under both Gaskell and Langley at the time they were engaged in their researches on this subject, and who had the opportunity of seeing the results gradually unfolded. It therefore occurred to me that it might be of interest if I gave you my impressions of those researches in the making, before turning to their subsequent clinical applications. For they stamped themselves deeply on my mind as a young man, and have greatly influenced the subsequent trend of my clinical ideas.

It is a curious and interesting fact that two such different characters as Gaskell and Langley, starting from such different standpoints, should have reached convergent and confirmatory results.

Gaskell was essentially a big man, alike in physique, personality and character. He poured out ideas with unstinted prodigality, often giving them to his pupils to develop and leaving them to take the credit. He delighted in sweeping generalisations in which, though they were sometimes based on inadequate detail, he was guided aright by his philosophic insight. He was above all an explorer of new fields. His work on the heart led him to examine the action of the nerves which went thereto, and this was the starting-point of his investigation of the sympathetic nervous system. I have often said that to read an account of this system before Gaskell is like reading an account of the circulation before Harvey. Both of these great observers reduced chaos to order. I will not weary you with details—to part of my audience they are well known; to the rest it can only be the broad deductions which will be of interest. Like all great discoveries, the basis was quite simple. He noted that the voluntary nerve fibres were of larger calibre than the involuntary ones. One set of these involuntary fibres leaves the central nervous system only between the great nerve plexuses which supply the arms and legs—this constitutes the sympathetic. The other set only arises above the nerve plexus to the arms and below that to the legs—this is called the parasympathetic. Whatever may be the ultimate destination of these fibres, their origin is always restricted to these areas. Whenever sympathetic and parasympathetic fibres are supplied to the same structure, their effects are antagonistic. The vertebrate body is fundamentally a tube within a tube, the inner tube being supplied by the smaller, and the outer mainly by the larger fibres. Extending his study to the nerves of sensation, he was able to divide the whole body into a series of segments, which in the head region had become complicated by the development of the brain. The deeper areas had a corresponding representation on the surface of the body; a generalisation which Sir Henry Head and Sir James Mackenzie applied brilliantly to the more accurate localisation of deep-seated disease. I must in passing emphasise how much of the conceptions of the nervous system I shall presently expound is owing to the combined experimental and clinical researches of Sir Henry Head, who even went so far as to offer his own body for experiment. He had the cutaneous nerves in his arm divided and then re-united in order to study the stages by which the venous sensations returned.

Gaskell was next led into a far more speculative field, the origin of the vertebrates. Many have deplored this diversion of his interest from a field in which he was supreme to one where he was at first relatively an amateur. It is not too much to say that morphologists actually resented his intrusion with revolutionary ideas into their preserves. It cannot be said that his views as to the origin of the vertebrates from an arthropod ancestor such as *Limulus* (the King Crab) command general acceptance, but we cannot lightly neglect the mass of evidence he accumulated in favour of his theory during the remaining years of his life. At first strongly prejudiced against it by my training in the morphological traditions of Frank Balfour, Lord Balfour's brilliant brother, so early cut off, I have gradually become more favourably disposed to it, as it was found to anticipate subsequent anatomical discoveries, and to provide a reasonable explanation of the origin of the system of ductless glands, a system which was little known when Gaskell first promulgated his theory.

Langley's starting-point was a different one. At first he was engrossed in the microscopic changes in glands during the process of secretion, particularly the storage of granules there as the forerunner of the characteristic secretion of the gland. This led him to study the nervous influences playing on such glands. In conjunction with Dickinson he discovered the paralysing influence of nicotine on the sympathetic nervous system and found that this was due to its breaking the connection just in front of the nerve cells in the sympathetic ganglia. He was quick to grasp the opportunity this gave him to unravel in detail the distribution of the sympathetic nerve fibres. Patiently, unremittingly, he laboured for years till the whole plan was clear. The splendid accuracy of Langley's mental microscope extended and completed the discoveries made by the great sweep of Gaskell's mental telescope. He was able to prove that the whole of the sympathetic system is planned to allow of wide and rapid diffusion of its effects.

When we come to study the effects of sympathetic stimulation, we find that primitively they served a preparation for fight or flight or for the expression of fright. They are all designed to activate the body for a struggle and to increase its powers of defence (Cannon). The pupil dilates to increase the perception of light; the heart beats more quickly and more forcibly to supply the muscles with blood; the blood vessels in the visceral area constrict, raising the blood pressure there, thus altering the distribution of blood and driving it from the digestive area, whose functions are simultaneously inhibited, into the skeletal and cardiac muscles, the lungs and the brain. The blood sugar is increased to supply fuel to the muscles.

The sweat glands are stimulated to cool the body heated by its excessive muscular effort and the hairs are erected in many animals to render them more alarming. Our own condition of "goose skin" is a persistence of this, though its occurrence singularly fails now to make us either look or feel more alarming. Some of our reflexes, like some of our structures, are vestigial.

The effects of parasympathetic stimulation are diametrically opposite to this; they serve for bodily conservation, replacing the display of kinetic energy by the storage of potential energy. As Cannon put it, to this group of nerves "belongs the quiet service of building up reserves and fortifying the body against times of need and stress".

Of these two great divisions then, the sympathetic is katabolic, directing the stream of energy outwards, while the parasympathetic is anabolic, directing the stream of energy inwards, where it is stored up. When one is stimulated into action, the other is checked.

The rhythm of life largely depends on the fluctuating balance between the sympathetic and parasympathetic. Thus fatigue following the expenditure of energy leads to sleep, when the parasympathetic gains control, and this arrest of external manifestations of energy lasts until the balance is restored in favour of the sympathetic, when we awaken again.

We see, therefore, that in pain, fear, rage and any intense excitement the anabolic activities of the body are in abeyance, and the katabolic activities go on unchecked. Potential energy is converted into kinetic, and reserves are freely spent. This is comprehensible since these katabolic activities are defensive in origin and aided the primitive animal in its struggle with its antagonist; and that complex organism the State, when at war, like the individuals of which it is composed, inhibits its anabolic activities, spends its reserves, and brings into play every katabolic activity which can aid it in its struggle for victory.

It may be asked, how, on this theory, is one

to account for the parasympathetic effects that are seen in overwhelming pain or fear, such as collapse and syncope? Rivers pointed out that a lowly organism has another method of defence—immobility—which takes the form in some animals of "shamming dead". Many animals, although able to perceive a moving object readily, seem to have little appreciation of a stationary one, so that immobility and preparation for fight or flight admit of no compromise. One or the other may be effective; to attempt to combine the two would be fatal. There must be either complete immobility through the parasympathetic, or violent action through the sympathetic. Thus confusion is avoided; if one comes into action the opposing group is inhibited.

It is abundantly clear that however the sympathetic nervous system is brought into action it, at any rate, simulates the ordinary expression of certain emotions, and pre-eminently the emotion of fear, such as palpitations, rapid action of the heart, sweating, blanched extremities, and gastro-intestinal disturbances. It is also clear that psycho-neurotics complain of physical symptoms of this type.

The primitive animal is geared up, as it were, ready to respond to danger through its sympathetic nervous system. Fear is a survival and often a perversion of that alertness of response. It is an instinct of enormous force in primitive man. Like the child, he feels surrounded by the unknown, and desires to come to terms with it. All religions pass through a God-fearing stage.

That many psychoneuroses are based on a repressed or subconscious fear is now clearly recognised. Fear, whether of evil spirits, of magic, or of the dark, panic fear dominated primitive man and, whenever our resistance is lowered by disease, by shock or by psychic conflict, we betray our ancestry. That strange primitive being, which lurks in the unconscious mind of us all, peeps out. We are certainly justified in stating that a condition of continued fear, whether recognised or not as such by the sufferer, is capable of producing the symptoms of which he so generally complains.

"Emotion moves us, hence the name", said Sherrington. It would perhaps be more accurate to say that it is designed to move us. When under conditions of modern life emotion is dissociated from the movement it should evoke under more primitive conditions, the sympathetic disturbance may continue. The mobilised army which is not allowed to fight the enemy becomes a danger to its own country.

Nervous impulses tend to run along accustomed channels. The exciting cause may long have passed from the realm of consciousness but its effects may continue. Designed for an intensive preparation for action or defence, the sympathetic response may be dissociated, perverted or prolonged, with serious effects on the individual. The pressure of the blood or its sugar content may be kept too high, the digestive processes in stomach or intestines may be inhibited, from purely emotional causes, yet ultimately leading to organic changes in structure.

You will observe that I am trying to establish the mechanism of the psychoneuroses on a biological basis. This was the aim and object of Rivers' later work.

W. H. R. Rivers was brought from Saint Bartholomew's Hospital to Cambridge by Michael Foster in 1893 to lecture on the physiology of the Special Senses. In 1898 an event occurred which was fraught with far-reaching consequences to English medicine. Yet it was not initiated by a medical man at all. It was Dr A. C. Haddon who organised an expedition to the Torres Straits and took Rivers, William McDougall and C. S. Myers with him. They went as physiologists; they returned as psychologists. This was in effect the beginning of the new psychology in England. McDougall's work in this respect has been accorded a wide and popular recognition. Myers has placed the study of industrial fatigue on a scientific basis. Rivers went specially to investigate the vision of uncivilised peoples. He came to the conclusion that while no substantial difference exists between the visual acuity of civilised and uncivilised peoples, the latter show a definite lack of colour discrimination. I believe that the Homeric poems show a similar lack. This suggests that much of colour perception is central rather than peripheral, psychological rather than physiological. It was extraordinarily fascinating to me to watch the evolution of Rivers from a physiologist, particularly concerned with the special senses, into an anthropologist, with a shrewd insight into the mentality of savages, based on a study of their sensory discrimination, and then into a psychotherapist. In my opinion, few were so well equipped to lay the foundations of a sane psychotherapy, for few psychotherapists had his biological training. In the treatment of war neuroses, Rivers found himself. His whole personality expanded as he grew to realise what was his true mission in life. I can bear personal testimony to his extraordinary influence in helping the shell-shocked soldier. Myers said, "He became another and a far happier man. Diffidence gave place to confidence, reticence to outspokenness, a somewhat laboured literary style to one remarkable for its ease and charm". Rivers himself said that after this war work "which brought me into contact with the real problems of life... I felt that it was impossible for me to return to my life of detachment". He found himself, and then, all too soon, we had to lose him. His untimely death in 1922 was a real disaster to English medicine.

The fundamental conception in Rivers' theory was an application and extension of Hughlings Jackson's great generalisation of the three layers of the central nervous system.

Hughlings Jackson regarded these three levels, reflex, sensori-motor and psychical, as representing successive stages in the development of the central nervous system, and maintained that in the disintegrative process of disease the highest, most recently acquired

35

levels, were the ones which would suffer first. Many symptoms of nervous disease were due to uncontrolled action of lower levels released from the restraint of higher levels. Rivers extended this conception by postulating a number of different layers, as it were, within the highest level. The development of the individual mind led to the formation of consecutive layers, each possessed of more reality-principle and self-control. But each individual started out equipped in these lower layers with earlier racial tendencies which were held more or less in abeyance by the higher layers. One might compare this part of the brain to that deep cleft in the rocks near Garavan, where for 100,000 years men dwelt, each generation merely living on the top of the débris left by its predecessors. And now, as excavations have removed layer after layer, more and more primitive types of man are revealed. Just so, in disease and in dreams this control of the higher layers is lessened and the older more primitive methods of thought reassert themselves. One can see, on this view, how natural it is for the sick person to revert to the primitive belief in magic.

Rivers did not accept Freud's conception of a censorship, but regarded the fantastic and symbolic forms in which hysteria and dreams manifest themselves as a regression to a lower level which was natural to the infantile stages of human development, individual or collective. He considered that a mental event could be relegated to the unconscious either by a conscious act of volition, in which case it could be recalled into consciousness, or by an "unwitting" suppression. This latter he regarded as a normal event in development and pointed out that it would be very inconvenient to the butterfly if it did not completely suppress the motor responses which had been of service to it when it was a caterpillar. Thus we reach the higher levels of our nervous system on the stepping stones not only of our dead selves, but of our long dead ancestors.

For the further elucidation of these problems

we must turn to the bio-chemical aspects. We may regard the ductless glands as a survival and specialisation of those chemical mechanisms by which an animal was controlled before a nervous system, as we know it, had been evolved. Hardly anything was known of this system when I was formerly in residence, though in 1891 G. R. Murray, one of our graduates, had begun to treat myxoedema and cretinism with thyroid extract, and this initiated a great advance in therapeutics. In 1894 Dr George Oliver, a physician practising in Harrogate, told Prof. Schäfer that he thought he had extracted a very active substance from the adrenal glands. Prof. Schäfer tested it and found that it both augmented the heart beat and raised the blood pressure. Some five years later Takamine prepared this active principle in a crystalline form and called it adrenalin. This was subjected to critical examination by T. R. Elliott in the physiological laboratory here, and Langley formulated a generalisation of far-reaching importance, i.e. the effect of adrenalin on any part is the same as the stimulation of the sympathetic nerve to that part. Now adrenalin is secreted by the adrenal medulla, and the cells composing this medulla are derived from sympathetic nerve ganglia. The principle of the wide diffusion of sympathetic impulses is here carried to a triumphant conclusion; the nervous effect is reinforced through the circulation by a chemical effect, which actually originates in sympathetic nerve cells.

Here we are on the very threshold of the mystery of the interrelations between nervous and chemical mechanisms. Gaskell had adumbrated this when he showed that the effects of nervous stimuli were metabolic in character, Langley and Elliott had both postulated a receptive substance at the nerve-ending where chemical changes occurred, and W. E. Dixon (whose death last year was such a blow to pharmacology) as long ago as 1907 showed that an actual chemical substance, now known to be a choline-ester, was formed in the heart when the vagus nerve to it was stimulated. In 1910 Dale began his work on this subject which has cleared up many of the difficulties surrounding it, particularly in relation to the capillary circulation.

But it is perhaps in the pituitary gland that we find this relationship between nervous and chemical mechanisms best emphasised. I have called this gland the leader in the endocrine orchestra. The anatomists of the past, looking at the brain encased in bone, and joined by a narrow stalk to this small pituitary body, also thus enclosed, like a brain in miniature, were struck by the idea of a little shrunken brain, which as it were, responded to or repeated the actions of the big brain above. Harvey Cushing, to whom more than to any other man our knowledge of the pituitary is due, recently gave a brilliant review of the relationship between this gland and the part of the brain known as the hypothalamus or diencephalon lying immediately above it; he re-echoed the saying of Ridley in 1695 that "It seems in a manner almost impossible to treat of one independently of the other". He went on to say: "No other single structure of the body is so doubly protected, so centrally placed, so well hidden [as the pituitary]. Here in this well-concealed spot, almost to be covered by a thumbnail, lies the very mainspring of primitive existence—vegetative, emotional and reproductive—on which with more or less success, man, chiefly, has come to superimpose a cortex of inhibitions. The symptoms arising from disturbance of this ancestral apparatus are beginning to stand out in their true significance. ...The diencephalon is an ancient part of the brain which remains essentially unaltered in all creatures that have a brain at all. Such primitive instincts as hunger, thirst and sleep also seem to be mediated through this region". Recent investigations show that this combined nervous and glandular apparatus is closely related to metabolic processes, to the primary emotions and to the sympathetic nervous system.

I will give you only one, and that a rather

amusing instance of the nervous and chemical relationships as seen in this gland. It is well known that if a cow dislikes a dairyman she can hold up her supply of milk. Leslie Pugh found that if he gave her an injection of pituitary extract she was quite unable to do this. Pituitrin seems necessary to start the flow of milk, and the cow's annoyance expressed itself by a nervous check on the secretion of this. Injecting pituitrin into the circulation rendered this emotional check nugatory, and the milk flowed once more.

Our knowledge of this part of the brain is mainly derived from two sources. No review of the influence of this school, however summary, can omit reference to the work of Charles Scott Sherrington who graduated here in 1883 and is now Waynflete Professor of Physiology at Oxford. Although most of his work has lain outside Cambridge, he is one of the most brilliant alumni of our school of physiology. His work on the integration of the nervous system is classical and has widely affected our conceptions of diseases of that system. The particular aspect of it relevant to my present topic is the demonstration that the destruction of the brain above the level of these basal ganglia does not prevent emotional expression but in point of fact allows of its more violent display. This has been confirmed clinically by studying the ravages wrought on human beings by lethargic encephalitis (sleepy sickness). There is something devilish about a disease that may alter the whole individuality emotionally and morally; which destroys Dr Jekyll and leaves only Mr Hyde. As we know, lethargic encephalitis specially affects the part of the brain just above the pituitary gland. It affords a striking illustration of Hughlings Jackson's dictum concerning the uncontrolled action of lower levels when released from the restraint of higher levels.

This then appears to be the plan on which the whole nervous system is built up. (1) A visceral level associated with the functions of organic life, with its head ganglion in the diencephalon

43

and closely associated with the more primitive chemical mechanisms of the ductless glands. Its action is widespread and tends to be explosive and emotionally uncontrolled. Immediately above this is (2) the mid-brain concerned with the statics and posture of the body; on the chemical side its action is more synthetic, acting through that great metabolic workshop, the liver. It receives sensory impressions from all over the body, sorts them out and sends them on to the next level above, which is (3) the sensori-motor level, and which is concerned with discriminative sensation and skilled voluntary movements. This level appears to be set free from chemical duties, so that it can specialise in these important functions. It acts largely in restraint of the lower levels. Lastly comes the highest psychical level. Here among other things we meet with a time sense, which enables us to "scorn delights and live laborious days" in pursuit of more ultimate benefits; while allowing the imaginative faculties to soar, it restrains their outward expression. Through it man, having laboriously acquired the power of speech, has to learn the still more subtle art of silence. To-day we hear much of the evil effects of repression, but it is noteworthy that each higher level of the nervous system inhibits the otherwise unrestrained action of the one immediately beneath it. That is where Rivers' subtle distinction between a pathological repression and suppression as a normal event comes in. But it is a distinction that many find hard to make, and a failure to make it spells psychoneurosis.

Modern medicine is, in fact, trying to reconcile two points of view which hitherto have seemed to be diametrically opposed. Van Helmont expressed this antinomy as long ago as 1617 in his doctrine of Blas and Gas. For him, Blas was an immaterial, intangible, spiritual force; while Gas, by which he meant carbonic-acid gas, or carbon dioxide which he discovered, typified chemical agencies. Van Helmont was, as Michael Foster recognised, a curious blending of the old and the new; on the one hand a patient, exact observer who had entered into the spirit of the new physics; on the other, a mystic, speculative dreamer. But he was three centuries ahead of his time in his view that disease was the failure of this Blas to govern aright, allowing germs to enter the body, thus bringing about chemical changes which it could not master. He grasped the cardinal idea of a sympathetic nervous system whereby the emotional state may influence resistance to disease. His term "Gas" has passed into everyday usage, but his "Blas" was lost sight of until the psychoneuroses of the war forced us to take a less materialistic view of medicine. But now his Blas is among us again to-day, puckish and elusive, wrapped in the garments of Adler, Jung and Freud, who, like Van Helmont, consider that the most important thing is to assist this spiritual force, this Blas, in overcoming the power of disease. Indeed, for some the "unconscious mind", of which we hear so much to-day, resides in the visceral nervous system, with its associated ductless glands. At any rate we are beginning to understand how a disagreeable thought can initiate an injurious chemical reaction or an alteration in the ductless glands may change the personality, while the severance of certain nervous tracts can place Prospero at the mercy of Caliban.

There is no break in the chain between the highest psychical functions and the visceral reflexes; there is the closest interaction between nervous and chemical mechanisms throughout. It is true that the sympathetic nervous system regulates our internal functions, while the sensori-motor nervous system keeps us in touch with the outside world, but it is also true that through the sympathetic we are geared up to deal with the more dramatic events in our environment. That the body acts as a whole both in health and disease is the important conclusion to be drawn. Lest it be thought that loyalty to this school may have led me to exaggerate its share in this work, let me quote from a recent work by Dr Cawadias, himself an Athenian Greek who was for some years in charge of the Therapeutical Clinic in the University of Paris. He says: "The British physiologists such as Foster, Gaskell, Langley, Sherrington, Schäfer, Bayliss, Starling and the American, Cannon—to quote only a few representative names—by demonstrating that man can no longer be considered as a bundle of organs or cells but as an integrated whole, gave the scientific basis of a synthetic conception of disease". It will be observed that the first four names on his list are those of Cambridge men of this period.

I hope, therefore, that I have been able to convey some idea of the part which Cambridge has played in this more vivid conception of the integration of the body, without appearing to claim too much as her share. For the freemasonry of science leads to such an interchange of ideas that it is as impossible as it is undesirable to be parochial in these matters.

On the other hand, it is obvious that consideration of time and space must lead to many omissions on my part. The space of my canvas has prevented me from dealing with the contributions of Hugh Anderson to neurology, especially on the nervous mechanisms of the eye. His later distinguished services as an administrator have tended to make men forget his earlier valuable researches. He was emphatically another man who found himself in Cambridge. I have said nothing of Roy who, primarily a physiologist with a genius for designing apparatus, founded the study of pathology here; nor of Kanthack who, alternating between my hospital and this school, brilliantly illuminated the general principles of pathology. Remembering the volume of his contributions to science, it is hard to realise that he was cut off at the early age of 35.

The time limitations which I laid down at the beginning exclude consideration of the splendid achievements of our bio-chemical school. I am always proud to remember that when Dr Sheridan Lea's health broke down in 1894, it fell to my lot and then to Dr Eichholz to keep physiological chemistry going here

until the great services of Sir Gowland Hop-
kins could be secured. But just this word on
that. His work on vitamins reinforces the lesson
of the hormones of the ductless glands—that
infinitesimal doses may produce profound
effects. As Starling said, every time we give a
dose of medicine we imply a belief that the
body can be influenced by chemical means and
we find justification for that belief in the fact
that the body manufactures chemical substances whereby to regulate itself. It is curious
that the most materialistic age in science should
have been the most sceptical as to the value of
drugs. When such a sceptic asked me how I
could imagine that 5 grs. of a drug could have
any effect on the whole body, I replied that the
body itself works with fractions of a milligram.

But drugs are but a fraction of medicine.
I have claimed in the past that the frontiers of
medicine are co-terminous with life. I am in-
clined to poach on the preserves of others and
claim that the term, the Humanities, is an apt
description of the medical sciences. Hippo-

crates adjured us to examine the whole of the patient. That involves a consideration of his whole attitude to life, the whole of his environment. For that task the widest possible education can hardly be wide enough. But at any rate, our aim here must be to give a humanistic trend to our student's scientific studies. He is going to practise an art and a science combined. I believe that in Cambridge we can provide him with the opportunities for equipping himself in both respects in a way that no mere technical training can do.

The difficulties we are passing through now are no new thing. In 1570, the Elizabethan Statutes made it no longer compulsory for medical students to take a degree in Arts or even to take a course of study in Arts before proceeding to the degree of Bachelor of Medicine. Consequently, medical graduates ceased to do so, with injurious effects on their general education. Since the war, we have been finding history repeating itself in this respect. We are at present engaged in an earnest attempt to overcome these difficulties, and I doubt not that we shall succeed. For Cambridge has always been adept at putting new wine into old bottles.

It is related of one of my·predecessors, John Gostlin, who was appointed Regius Professor of Physic in 1623, that his joy at returning to Cambridge was "almost excessive". I trust that the higher levels of my nervous system may prevent me from any unseemly manifestation of my own joy. Moreover, it is indeed a sobering thought for anyone to realise that he has to follow such men as Paget, Allbutt and Rolleston. Nevertheless, I will admit that it is a great joy to return to the place that has coloured the whole of my subsequent life. I came here the first time, shy, awkward and diffident, to meet with the most kindly encouragement; what germs of promise my teachers cunningly detected, they assiduously cultivated. I return, filled with the desire to repay something of the debt I owe to Cambridge.

Milton Keynes UK
Ingram Content Group UK Ltd.
UKHW032321161024
449665UK00001B/2